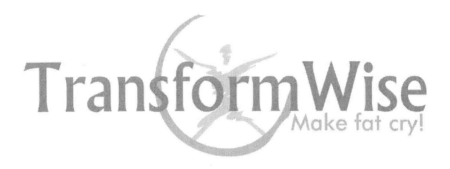

TransformWise
Your Complete Guide to a Wise Body Transformation

Dr. Scott A. Johnson

Scott A. Johnson

TransformWise: your complete guide to a wise body transformation / Scott A. Johnson

ISBN 1493652362

ISBN 978-1493652365

Discover more books by Scott A. Johnson at authorscott.com

Printed by CreateSpace, an Amazon.com Company

Scott A. Johnson

DISCLAIMERS OF WARRANTY AND LIMITATION OF LIABILITY
The author provides all information on an "as is" and "as available" basis. Author makes no representations or warranties of any kind, expressed or implied, as to the information, materials or products mentioned.

Always consult a qualified medical professional before beginning any nutritional or exercise program and seek the advice of your physician with any questions you may have regarding any medical condition. The information contained in this book is for educational and informational purposes only and not meant to replace medical advice, diagnosis or treatment in any manner. Never delay or disregard professional medical advice. Use the information solely at your own risk, the author accepts no responsibility for the use thereof.

The Food and Drug Administration (FDA) has not evaluated the statements contained in this book or associated materials. The information and materials are not meant to diagnose, prescribe, or treat any disease, condition, illness or injury.

USE AT YOUR OWN RISK
By voluntarily undertaking any exercise or nutritional guidance contained in this e-book or supportive materials, you assume any and all risk of injury, loss or damage suffered. The author disclaims liability for incidental or consequential damages and assumes no responsibilities for loss or damages suffered as a result of the use or misuse of any information or content associated with this e-book and supportive materials.

Scott A. Johnson

TABLE OF CONTENTS

Scott A. Johnson

FOREWORD

Did you ever decide to lose some weight but you just couldn't do it or maintain it over a period of time? You might just find the answer in this new book by Scott Johnson. "TransformWise" takes a holistic approach to weight loss. Changing your diet without considering a good exercise program or the other way around will not work in the long run and might just put you on the endless carousel of yo-yo dieting which will ultimately damage your metabolism. The solution to weight loss is more complicated than just counting calories. This book will give a good explanation of some of the processes in your body and why it is important to take a holistic "life-style change" approach to weight loss. Scott Johnson will walk you through a no non-sense approach to nutrition and explain how good nutrition and portion sizes should be part of any weight loss attempt.

He will also show you why weight loss is not simply the result of calories in versus calories out. Your body produces many hormones that are very tightly linked to fat accumulation as well as fat loss. This is the reason why it is difficult for an obese person to just eat less, lose weight and then keep it off over an extended period of time. Every fat cell for example is busy producing hormones that will affect the way the body is working. Several weight-related hormones are also produced in the lining of the intestinal tract and influence how your neurotransmitters in the brain are activated or deactivated. Hunger center and satiety center in the brain can both be activated or inhibited depending on how these hormones rise and fall. Scott Johnson explains these very complicated interactions in a simple and understandable way. Nutrition is not just adding fuel in form of sugars, protein, and fat to the body, food choices also directly influence the way our genes are decoded by the cells. The food you eat will tell the cells how to work and therefore influence multiple functions and pathways in the body. We call this the field of nutrigenomics or food-related epigenetics.

But nutrition and food choices are only a part of the equation when it comes to a holistic approach to weight loss. Like food, exercise is able to change the way your cells are working. Exercise itself is of course a calorie burning activity, but it's equally important that over time beneficial epigenetic changes are initiated by exercise. Over time, you will lose fat and gain muscle mass which in turn will increase your basic metabolic rate, the amount of calories you are burning in 24 hours at rest. A lot has been written about exercise and what might be best: aerobic versus anaerobic, short versus long, hard versus light and so on. Recent scientific evidence suggests that we use Metabolic Resistance Training as a good form of fat-reducing exercise. In this book you'll learn what this form of exercise is, why you should look into this and why the recovery after exercise plays such an important role.

Finally you will be guided through the necessary equipment and exercises to get you closer to your goal of losing weight and sustaining a healthy body mass index. The exercise suggestions will take into account whether you are a beginner, intermediate, or advanced exerciser and select the exercises accordingly.

I highly recommend this book. It is very well written and based on scientific evidence. I am sure that it will help you on your quest for a better life and body weight.

Olivier Wenker, MD, MBA, DEAA, ABAARM
Professor of Anesthesiology and Perioperative Medicine, The University of Texas
Fellow in Integrative Oncology, American Academy of Antiaging and Regenerative Medicine
Editor-in-chief, The Internet Journal of Nutrition and Wellness
International Keynote Speaker and Member of the Scientific Advisory Council for Young Living Essential Oils

Scott A. Johnson

CHAPTER 1

The Value of Eating Better

Let's face it; eating a health-promoting diet isn't easy in today's world full of oversized portions, sugar-laced desserts, and fast food restaurants on every corner. You, the consumer, are bombarded with advertisements for unhealthy foods, which when consumed cause the release of "feel good" chemicals like dopamine, creating a greater desire for these foods. Some foods even have chemicals or ingredients added to them that make them more addicting.

Obesity and overweight trends worldwide demonstrate the harmful effects these trends have had on societies. Diseases associated with carrying extra pounds—heart disease, diabetes, metabolic syndrome, osteoarthritis, depression and cancer—are growing at alarming rates. Unfortunately, these poor eating habits are being passed on to the next generation perpetuating this cycle of ill health among our children. In fact, the obesity epidemic is such a large problem that David S. Ludwig, MD, PhD, a pediatrician and researcher at Children's Hospital Boston and Harvard professor stated "Obesity is such that this generation of children could be the first in the history of the United States to live less healthful and shorter lives than their parents."

Governments and health care professionals are scrambling to slow or reverse these trends through informational campaigns, tough legislation and sometimes extreme policies. One such attempt to promote healthy eating was the release of My Plate by the United States Department of Agriculture. While this program is a good starting point, it falls short of the comprehensive guidance required to truly eat better. The TransformWise approach to eating is intended to expound what eating better means in a simple and straightforward manner, and provide the knowledge to implement proven strategies to improve your health and well-being.

You are what you eat is very literal—some of you are conjuring up pictures of French fries, donuts and hamburgers. What you eat supplies your body the nutrients and building blocks that are essential to optimal health and well-being. Your body breaks down the "fuel" (food) you supply so that it can maintain numerous physiological functions necessary for life. Supplying your body with junk food and unhealthy options is the equivalent of putting regular unleaded fuel in a NASCAR race car. The car will run on this fuel, but it will not be performing optimally and eventually the knocking caused by the wrong octane level may lead to damage. You simply can't expect to put the wrong food into your body consistently and expect to perform your best, nor can you expect to avoid the negative long-term consequences to your health.

Conversely, when you supply your body with abundant quantities of nutrient dense foods—fruits and vegetables, healthy fats, lean protein, wholesome carbohydrates, and plenty of water—you provide the optimal environment for your cells to thrive. When you have healthy cells you have healthy tissues, healthy organs and organ systems that thrive, ultimately leading to the optimal state of health known as vigor and vitality. Now, don't get me wrong, this doesn't mean you will never get sick, or that you will avoid disease altogether, but it does limit your risk for these adverse conditions.

Beyond limiting your risk of illness and disease, healthy eating provides a variety of benefits to your overall well-being, allowing you to live a more fulfilling and healthy life.

Maintain a healthy weight. When you eat the right foods you are more likely to maintain a healthy weight or lose weight if you so desire. Diets rich in fiber and protein have been shown to help individuals achieve and maintain a healthy weight. Drinking enough water can accelerate your metabolism. And replacing empty calories—high calorie foods with little or no nutrients—with healthy choices improves your calorie to energy expenditure ratio.

Feel Better. Fruits and vegetables are loaded with nutrients that provide sustainable energy levels to help you accomplish what you need to during the day. Supplying your body with the right amount of healthy nutrients also influences your mood, making it easier to maintain a balanced emotional state, and manage stress and negative emotions. By flooding your body with a steady stream of these nutrients you are more likely to realize true vigor and vitality, enjoy sustainable energy levels, experience abundant physical strength and maintain a balanced mood and emotions.

Maximize cognitive functioning. No one wants to experience a decline in brain or cognitive functioning, and nutrition is the most important factor for staying mentally sharp. Key nutrients are essential for your brain to perform at its best including omega-3 fatty acids—particularly DHA, vitamin B12, iron, antioxidants and other phytonutrients. Many nutrients—like those found in berries—protect brain neurons and enhance neuroplasticity, or the ability of the brain to form new neural connections throughout life in response to new behaviors, information or sensory stimulation. Feed your brain healthy options and optimum health is more likely.

Look your best. Eating better, combined with regular physical activity, helps you achieve and maintain your ideal physique. Your hair, nails and skin will all benefit as they take advantage of the flood of beneficial nutrients that eating better supplies. Everyone has an inner splendor waiting to be revealed and the TransformWise approach to eating can help you reveal it. Discovering your ideal physique also does wonders for your self-confidence. When you look your best you don't mind being in public, even if it's in your swimsuit.

Improve sleep quality. Your diet directly influences sleep quality. Some foods—caffeine, coffee, tea, high-fat foods—increase nervous system activity or cause the release of hormones that prevent a restful night's sleep. Conversely, healthy foods like cherries, almonds, bananas, and oatmeal calm your nervous system and trigger the release of sleep-inducing hormones, making it more likely you will sleep peacefully.

Balance your mood. Have you ever been around someone who is really hungry? Chances are they weren't a very pleasant person to hang out with. Healthy foods release nutrients more slowly and sustainably, allowing your brain to utilize these nutrients to help balance your mood. Moreover, eating better influences the release of neurotransmitters—particularly serotonin—that helps balance mood.

Provide your body the right foods and realize your best healthy self today.

CHAPTER 2

Meal Frequency, When More is Better

The typical eating pattern of individuals includes three meals—breakfast, lunch and dinner. However, scientific research suggests that this is not the healthiest eating pattern for optimal human health. This entrenched paradigm may be contributing to the ill health of millions including obesity, heart disease and diabetes. Consuming three meals a day with large gaps between each meal disrupts your energy and hormone balance, slows down your metabolism, leads to rapid spikes and drops in blood sugar levels and even negatively affects cholesterol levels (1-7).

It is well-known that elevated cholesterol levels are a risk factor for cardiovascular disease. Moreover, a slow metabolism can lead to overweight and obesity. And postprandial hyperglycemia—elevated blood sugar levels following a meal—is highly associated with cardiovascular disease (8-9), and is an indication that a person has or may be at risk for developing type II diabetes.

In order to avoid this roller coaster of blood sugar and hormone levels and decrease cholesterol accumulation, it is wise to consume five to six small, well-balanced meals per day. This may seem counterintuitive to some, that eating more will actually aid weight management and overall health. However, the key here is small, well-balanced meals based on your body size not a figure that only meets the nutritional requirements of the few. And available scientific research supports eating smaller, more frequent meals.

A 1993 study that included 19 men and women with normal cholesterol levels were divided into two groups. One group ate the standard three meals per day, while the other group consumed nine smaller meals per

15

day, with no difference among the groups in macronutrient intake. Interestingly, the scientists found that the group consuming nine meals per day experienced decreased low-density lipoprotein (LDL) levels, also known as bad cholesterol, and maintained a more consistent level of glucose in the blood (10). This confirmed the findings of an earlier two-week study involving seven men, which concluded that increasing meal frequency has a positive effect on total cholesterol levels and serum insulin levels (11).

An even larger study was completed at the University of California from 1984 to 1987 that included 2034 men and women aged 50 to 89. Again researchers reported lower total cholesterol levels among those consuming more frequent meals, without an increase in calories, when compared to those eating fewer meals (12). This cholesterol reduction was consistent even after adjusting for smoking, alcohol, waist-to-hip ratio, systolic blood pressure, body mass index and dietary nutrients.

Beyond helping to reduce total cholesterol and rapid surges and declines in blood sugar, meal frequency also effects hormone balance (13), thermogenesis and appetite control. Research suggests that eating more frequent meals revs up metabolism and thermogenesis in healthy obese women (14)—when your body uses excess calories to produce heat rather than storing them as fat. Two additional studies found a positive effect on post meal thermogenesis and fat utilization (15, 16).

One of the challenges with the three meals per day approach is the long fasting period between meals. Increasing meal frequency reduces fasting time between meals and studies suggest this helps control and curb appetite (17-19).

Sample eating plans with increased meal frequency:

Six Meals and Snacks
7:00 a.m. – Breakfast
10:00 a.m. – Healthy Snack
12:00 p.m. – Lunch
3:00 p.m. – Healthy Snack
5:30 p.m. – Dinner
8:00 p.m. – Healthy snack

Five Meals and Snacks
7:00 a.m. – Breakfast
10:00 a.m. – Healthy Snack
12:30 p.m. – Lunch
3:30 p.m. – Healthy Snack
6:00 p.m. – Dinner

CHAPTER 3

Sensible Meals and Portions

The perfect, one-size-fits-all diet doesn't exist—despite the well-intentioned efforts of many who try to design such a program. The fact is, each person is biologically unique and therefore will require different nutrients, portion sizes. etc. One of the keys to healthy eating is to listen to your body. Do you have digestive problems after consuming certain foods? Or do you feel worse after eating a particular food? Your body's response to the foods you eat can be an invaluable guide to what you should and shouldn't eat. That being said, there are a few guiding principles and effective strategies that may help you eat better, always adjusting to your individual body needs.

Portion sizes have ballooned out of control, as have the waistlines of countless individuals worldwide. The portions divvied out of many common foods and beverages today have doubled and even tripled the number of calories provided when compared to 20 years ago. Combine this with a more sedentary lifestyle and it is no wonder so many people worldwide are overweight or obese. Some simple steps can help you eat reasonable portion sizes: share a restaurant meal, use small or medium plates instead of large plates and fill your plate half full of vegetables to leave less room for the less healthy items.

Eating a sensible portion can be challenging when all you have to compare to is oversized portions. However, a simple approach is to use your hand as a guide—this makes portion sizes more proportional to your size and caloric needs. For example, to create a reasonably portioned meal the following would be sensible:
~ a serving of protein that fits in the palm of your hand
~ a serving of fruits and vegetables covering your entire open hand
~ a serving of wholesome carbohydrates that fit inside your cupped hand

~ and a small serving of fat about the size of your thumb

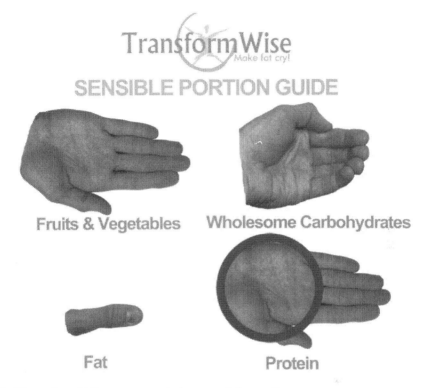

This TransformWise approach to sensible portions ensures a reasonably portioned and well-balanced meal based on your body size. You can also use it as a guide to balance your snacks, particularly focusing on metabolic balancing, to avoid the hormone and blood sugar roller coaster that can occur when eating an unbalanced meal, and to encourage satiety.

Now, before you go out and start filling your hand with these portions, we need to discuss what constitutes healthy choices, so you actually eat better, not just the right portions.

Vegetables and fruits should make up the bulk of your diet, aiming for 6 to 12 servings daily. Choose fruits and vegetables in their whole, natural, and unprocessed state whenever possible to ensure maximum nutrient density. Processing such as making applesauce out of apples or orange juice out of oranges can deplete essential nutrients and enzymes diminishing the value of these nutrient-dense, wholesome carbohydrates. Choose local, organic produce that is in season to avoid pesticides and other harmful chemicals and to obtain maximum nutritional value. Eat a wide variety of fruits and vegetables that includes all the colors of the rainbow. Each of the wonderful colors you see in produce identifies a beneficial nutrient, such as beta-carotene in carrots and anthocyanins in blueberries.

Wholesome carbohydrates should be chosen over refined carbohydrates and even complex carbohydrates. Fruits and vegetables are definitely wholesome carbohydrates, but separating them from other carbs helps us see the importance of making fruits and vegetables the center of our eating plan. Many of the high-quality protein sources are also carbs, such as quinoa, beans and legumes. Complex carbohydrates are often thought of as a healthy option, but depending on how a chocolate cake is made, it too could be considered a complex carbohydrate. This is why wholesome carbohydrates, like whole grain einkorn wheat, whole grain oats, brown rice, whole grain kamut pasta and brown rice pasta, are suggested and a better definition.

Protein should come from high-quality and lean sources, such as fish, turkey, chicken, 95 percent lean grass-fed beef, beans, legumes, nuts and seeds—particularly quinoa, which is a seed, not a grain as popularly believed. Protein promotes satiety, helping you to eat less. The Institute of Medicine recommends adults consume a minimum of 0.8 grams of protein per 2.2 pounds of body weight just to avoid breaking down your own tissues for energy. Those who are more active and athletes will need to consume even more protein (1.25 to 1.75 grams per 2.2 pounds).

Fat has an undeserved bad reputation due to years of "food experts" advocating its avoidance. However, fat is a necessary nutrient that plays a vital role in your health and, when added to a meal, acts as a metabolic regulator. In other words, it helps decrease spikes in blood sugar and hormones following a meal, which leads to better appetite control and accelerated fat burning potential. What's crucial is the type of fats and the ratio of unhealthy to healthy fats you consume. Preferred sources of fat include marine oils (omega-3 fatty acids), olive oil, coconut oil, avocados and sunflower oil. Trans fats and partially-hydrogenated oils, found in fast food and many baked and fried goods, should be avoided, while saturated fat should be limited.

The average adult human body consists of 50 to 75 percent **water**, making it the most abundant component found in your body. Your body will not function optimally without ideal hydration. Water helps flush out toxins, transports nutrients to your cells and provides a moist environment for body tissues. Every day, water is lost through perspiration, respiration, urination and bowel movements, and must be replenished through food and drink.

The old axiom to drink eight, eight-ounce glasses of water per day is another attempt at a one-size-fits-all standard. A more practical approach to water consumption is to personalize your daily water intake to your current state of health and body size. A simple way to achieve this is by drinking half of your body weight in ounces each day. For example, a 120 pound woman would drink 60 ounces of water each day. Clean filtered water is the preferred choice for hydration because alcohol, soda and other high-sugar beverages can actually deplete your water storage and harm your health.

Drinking sufficient water is essential for your body transformation to occur. Even mild dehydration can slow your metabolism by up to three percent. Conversely, drinking ample amounts of clean water can rev up your metabolism. In fact, a December 2003 study published in *The Journal of Clinical Endocrinology and Metabolism* found that drinking 17 ounces of water at one time increases metabolism by an average of 30 percent only 10 minutes following consumption.

Increased water consumption also has a balancing effect on your appetite. By ingesting proper amounts of water, you feel fuller helping to control your appetite. Finally, water is needed to build your body, serving to energize every cell and organ in the body.

Now that we have a better understanding of what we should eat, let's discuss a few items that can hamper your body transformation.

High-fructose corn syrup (HFCS) - While all added sugars should be limited as much as possible, HFCS is particularly harmful. HFCS is a sweetener created by processing corn sugar to increase the level of fructose to about 55 percent. It is rapidly absorbed causing an equally rapid spike in blood sugar. Research suggests that your body doesn't process HFCS like regular sugar (sucrose), which means it doesn't shut off your appetite center, causing you to overeat. Your liver must convert HFCS to glucose, but when too much HFCS is consumed it gets stored as fat, contributing to obesity and fatty liver deposits. In addition, HFCS increases triglyceride levels, LDL cholesterol levels, contributes to diabetes and metabolic syndrome, depresses your immune system and even accelerates the aging process. *Commonly found in: soda/soft drinks, baked goods, candy, sauces, salad dressings, yogurt, cereals. Other names: glucose-fructose syrup, isoglucose.*

Monosodium glutamate (MSG) - MSG is a flavor enhancer added to thousands of foods commonly consumed every day. It is highly associated with short-term reactions such as headache, flushing, numbness or burning in the face and neck area, heart palpitations, nausea, chest pain, difficulty breathing and weakness. MSG overstimulates the glutamine receptors in the brain, which enhances salty and sweet flavors. Some reports suggest that this overexcitement of glutamine receptors can cause cell death or damage and eventually declined cognitive function. *Commonly found in: Chinese food, canned vegetables, soups, processed meats, crackers, frozen dinners, chicken and beef broths, potato chips. Other names: autolyzed yeast, calcium caseinate, gelatin, glutamate, glutamic acid, hydrolyzed protein, hydrolyzed vegetable protein, monopotassium glutamate, sodium caseinate, textured protein, yeast extract, yeast food, yeast nutrient.*

Trans fats - Trans fats are a man-made fat used to enhance the flavor of and extend the shelf life of many foods. Research suggests it is more harmful than saturated fat and devastating to the cardiovascular system. Trans fats increase LDL cholesterol and triglyceride levels while lowering HDL cholesterol levels, which significantly increases the risk of heart disease, heart attack and stroke. It is also associated with an increased risk of developing type II diabetes. *Commonly found in: fried foods, baked goods, potato chips, crackers, margarine, fast food, packaged foods, cookies, frozen foods, dips. Other names: partially hydrogenated vegetable oil.*

Sodium nitrite - A salty preservative used in some meats, sodium nitrite has been linked to certain cancers and heart disease. Research suggests that those who eat the most processed meat (known to contain sodium nitrite) have a greater risk of cancer and heart disease than people who eat red meat. During digestion, this ingredient combines with amino acids to form nitrosamines, which are very harmful to the liver and pancreas and highly carcinogenic. *Commonly found in: Processed meats, hot dogs, sausage, bacon, beef jerky, deli meats, canned soups. Other names: sodium nitrate.*

Artificial sweeteners - Artificial sweeteners are used in a variety of products to decrease caloric intake. However, evidence suggests that diet soda drinkers are more likely to become overweight, obese and have a larger waistline than those who drink full sugar soft drinks. Beyond obesity, artificial sweeteners are associated with an increased risk of heart disease, diabetes, metabolic syndrome and kidney disorders. Some reports indicate that artificial sweeteners may cause gastrointestinal problems, allergic reactions, migraines, cancer, and kidney, liver and thyroid damage. *Commonly found in: Soft drinks/soda, sugar-free gum, candy, yogurt, diet foods, many foods labeled sugar-free, snack bars, cereal. Other names: acesulfame potassium, aspartame, neotame, saccharin, sucralose, malitol, erythritol, isomalt, lactitol, hydrogenated starch, hydrolysate.*

Unfortunately, the **wheat** of today is not the wholesome and beneficial wheat of our ancestors. In an effort to improve yield and make wheat more pesticide resistant man genetically modified (GM) wheat resulting in changes in the way wheat affects humans biologically. Today's GM wheat promotes excess inflammation, causes skin problems, promotes obesity, increases the body's acidity, disrupts the digestive system, spikes insulin levels, rapidly increases blood sugar levels and is a factor in autoimmune disorders. With the exception of einkorn wheat, which is ancient wheat that has avoided tampering by man, most wheat products should be limited or avoided, particularly if you have diabetes, an autoimmune disorder or excess inflammation. Besides einkorn, sprouted breads, quinoa and amaranth are good substitutes.

In addition to the above it is wise to reduce or eliminate soda (even diet), genetically modified organisms (GMO) products, sweets, alcohol, stimulants – caffeinated products, coffee and tea, or any other addictive harmful substance.

It should be noted that when changing your diet, particularly if it is a drastic change, you may experience temporary symptoms such as headache, stomachache, nausea and overall reduced feeling of wellness as your body adapts.

Scott A. Johnson

Meal and Snack Recommendations/Ideas:

Breakfast –
~ Oatmeal with raisins; pears and cottage cheese
~ Oatmeal with blueberries and Greek yogurt
~ Oatmeal with honey, pears and almonds
~ Berry Spinach Smoothie
~ Nut Butter Spinach Smoothie
~ Egg omelet with peppers, onions, mushrooms, black beans and goat cheese; peach
~ Oatmeal blueberry pancakes; scrambled eggs
~ Whole-grain peanut butter and banana waffles

Lunch or Dinner –
~ Spinach salad with grilled chicken breast, raspberries and pecans
~ Mixed greens with salmon, grapefruit sections, pistachios and avocado; balsamic vinaigrette
~ Spinach and mixed greens with mixed berries, pecans, tomatoes and pan-seared chicken breast; vinegar and olive oil dressing
~ Turkey, cranberry, Swiss cheese and avocado Panini (whole wheat); steamed or raw mixed vegetables and hummus
~ Pan-seared chicken breast; brown rice; steamed or raw mixed vegetables and hummus
~ Grilled chicken quesadilla (whole wheat tortilla) with black beans, goat cheese and cilantro; roasted asparagus
~ Sautéed chicken over brown rice topped with olives, peppers, garlic and red onion; pineapple with Greek yogurt
~ Baked salmon; steamed vegetables; sprouted grain roll with butter
~ Vegetable curry over brown rice
~ Baked sweet potato with cinnamon and butter; mixed greens, blue cheese, blueberries, apple slices and pecans with raspberry vinaigrette
~ Tilapia and quinoa; roasted vegetables
~ Herb roasted salmon with roasted new potatoes; mixed greens with balsamic vinaigrette
~ Kamut pasta with tomato sauce; garlic, parmesan green beans
~ Salsa chicken tortilla salad

AM or PM Snack –
~ Apples and peanut butter
~ Apples and cheese
~ Celery and peanut butter

~ Pears and cottage cheese
~ Pear, peach, banana, or apple with a handful of nuts
~ Nuts and dried cranberries
~ Mixed berries in Greek yogurt
~ Raspberries and Greek yogurt with honey
~ Fruits or nuts with 70% cacao dark chocolate
~ Fruit and nut snack bar (my favorite is Young Living Essential Oils' Slique Bar)
~ Carrots, broccoli and cauliflower with roasted garlic cream cheese
~ Carrots, broccoli and cauliflower with hummus
~ Carrots, broccoli and cauliflower with white bean dip
~ Pea pods and string cheese
~ Sliced tomato with feta cheese and olive oil
~ Edamame with olive oil and lemon
~ Avocado
~ Turkey jerky
~ Tuna fish on sprouted grain crackers
~ Roasted asparagus and hardboiled egg
~ Dried fruit and pistachios
~ Olives
~ Seed, nut and dried fruit mix

Eating better doesn't mean you can never get to have a treat or dessert, but it does mean remembering the last time you did have them. In order to maximize fat lass and optimize your well-being it is recommended that no more than three desserts or treats are consumed each week, with a cupped hand being the general serving size. Great alternatives to desserts or sugary snacks are dried fruit, peanut butter with honey, fruit with yogurt dip and dark chocolate.

CHAPTER 4

The Emotional and Hormone Connection to Transforming

Hormones are vital chemical messengers that influence virtually every cell, organ and function of the body, and even a minor imbalance in any one of the known hormones can wreak havoc on your vigor and vitality. Hormones are highly involved in weight loss, including metabolism, appetite and where fat is stored in the body. Frankly, any book providing guidance to transform your body or discover optimal health would be incomplete without discussing the role of hormones.

In an over simplistic view, body transformation requires expending more calories than you consume. But this thinking misses a key factor in achieving rapid, sustainable results—hormone and emotional balance. For genuine transformation to occur the dynamic relationship between eating, movement, hormones and even genetics has to be considered. In other words you must take a holistic approach.

Just the very act of attempting to lose weight or increase your activity level after being sedentary can be stressful and increase the release of hormones like cortisol that sabotage your transformation efforts. Cortisol is involved in blood pressure regulation, kidney function, glucose control, muscle building and the breakdown and storage of fat. A delicate balance of cortisol must exist for transformation and vitality to be present because an insufficient level disrupts metabolism and other essential body processes, whereas an excess levels is associated with a growing list of adverse health outcomes—obesity, metabolic syndrome, depression, impaired immune system function and more.

Cortisol is released by the adrenal glands signaling the body to breakdown fats and carbohydrates to provide your body with the required energy to respond when your body experiences stress or a stressor. When stress levels return to normal, cortisol stimulates your appetite to replenish the fats and carbohydrates utilized during the stress response. Chronically elevated cortisol levels intensify feelings of hunger, especially for high-calorie, fatty and sugary foods that supply high quantities of energy. In addition, cortisol encourages fat to be stored in the abdominal area.

Insufficient cortisol can be equally damaging, disrupting metabolism, causing fatigue, excessively low blood pressure and may even lead to Addison's Disease—a condition where the adrenal glands do not produce enough of the hormones cortisol and aldosterone, leading to muscle weakness, fatigue, low blood pressure and skin discoloration.

To optimize cortisol levels, one must properly manage stress, exercise, get adequate and consistent sleep and eat a balanced diet. In addition, adaptogenic herbs like ashwagandah, ginseng and schizandra, essential oils like cedarwood and lavender, and nutrients like vitamin C, B-complex, L-theanine and 5-HTP (5-Hydroxytryptophan) naturally optimize cortisol levels

Recently researchers have discovered that cortisol has a partner in crime when it comes to storing abdominal fat—11-beta-hydroxysteroid-dehydrogenase, or HSD. A catalyzing enzyme, HSD amplifies cortisol exposure by converting the inactive form of cortisol—cortisone—back to the active form, encouraging fat storage in the abdominal cavity.

Another important hormone, ghrelin, controls hunger signals. It is produced in your stomach and sends signals to the brain when you are hungry. Reducing calories increases the production of ghrelin, and research suggests that it can take up to 12 months for your ghrelin levels to reset, meaning your brain is constantly receiving hunger signals. Fortunately, intense physical activity helps decrease ghrelin levels (20) making exercise intensity one of the biggest keys to losing weight.

A hormone released from fat cells, leptin is key to energy expenditure and intake. It sends signals to your brain that influence how many calories you eat and how many you burn. Your body releases more leptin if you have more fat cells, but if too much fat is present in the body, your brain stops responding properly to leptin, a condition called leptin resistance. Weight loss enhances leptin sensitivity. Indeed, the more weight you lose the greater your sensitivity to leptin. Animal studies also suggest that exercise may increase leptin sensitivity, thus offering appetite suppression (21-23).

Adiponectin is also released from fat cells; however, unlike leptin the leaner your body is the more of it you release. It also suppresses appetite, boosts your metabolism and triggers fat burning. In addition it increases your muscle's ability to use carbohydrates for energy. Researchers have discovered that exercise increases adiponectin levels, leading to improved weight loss and body composition (24-26). Emerging research suggests that marine omega 3 fatty acids moderately increase adiponectin levels (27).

Decreased insulin sensitivity means your cells require greater amounts of insulin to move excess glucose out of the bloodstream. Just as meal frequency influences insulin sensitivity, exercise also positively influences insulin sensitivity, which is important for muscle building and exercise recovery. Too many of the wrong carbohydrates can rapidly raise blood sugar levels, increasing the storage of fat and preventing fat cells from releasing fat for energy. It is a well-known fact that exercise improves insulin sensitivity, particularly longer bouts of exercise (28). One study found that exercising after fasting, such as first thing in the morning before eating, improves insulin sensitivity and muscle composition (29).

Glucagon is a hormone produced by the pancreas, which is responsible for the breakdown and release of stored fats and carbohydrates for energy usage. It acts the opposite of insulin, however, when equal amounts of insulin and glucagon are present in the blood stream, insulin wins out and will perform its function. Primarily released between meals and during exercise, glucagon can also be increased by eating a protein-rich, low carbohydrate meal.

Human growth hormone (HGH) is critical to normal growth and development and influences cell reproduction and regeneration. It is vital that you optimize HGH levels to achieve the body transformation you desire. Optimized HGH levels increase the synthesis of protein, and aid muscle growth, recovery and repair. It is also involved in fat metabolism, bone health and energy production. Exercise stimulates the release of HGH, which improves body composition by decreasing body fat and increasing lean muscle (30-31). Available scientific research suggests that higher intensity exercise increases circulating growth hormone better than low-intensity exercise (32, 33).

Exercise, particularly interval training, boosts levels of epinephrine, more commonly known as adrenaline, a hormone that has been found to increase fat and carbohydrate breakdown for energy production. Elevated levels of epinephrine increase heart rate, muscle strength and blood pressure to prepare the body for strenuous activity.

The hormone peptide cholecystokinin (CCK) aids digestion by stimulating the release of digestive enzymes from the pancreas and bile salts from the gallbladder. It also promotes satiety sooner and increases the duration of fullness so you experience longer periods of time without feeling hungry. Scientists believe this is due to CCK's ability to slow gastric emptying rates (34, 35).

Among women, too much estrogen slows metabolism and leads to excess storage of fat in the hip and abdominal area. On the other hand, balanced estrogen levels aid weight loss by influencing enzymatic activity, specifically that of lipoprotein lipase (LPL) and hormone sensitive lipase (HSL), and helps determine where fat is stored. LPL decreases fat absorption within cells, while HSL helps regulate fat metabolism. Interestingly, HSL activity peaks during exercise, triggering the breakdown of fat. Women naturally have more subcutaneous fat than men and the preferred storage site of fat in a woman's body is the hips, thighs and buttocks. During menopause, when estrogen levels decline, fat storage in these areas accelerates.

Progesterone balances out estrogen and when too little is present estrogen dominance occurs. Progesterone influences metabolism, decreases insulin, supports thyroid function, facilitates the utilization of stored fat for energy needs and helps control appetite. Balancing both estrogen and progesterone is critical to the overall well-being of women, however, synthetic estrogens are highly associated with cancer and heart disease. Natural bioidentical hormones are the best solution to this problem. These hormones possess the same molecular structure as the hormones your body produces on its own.

Testosterone is as important in body transformation for men as estrogen is for women. Balanced testosterone levels are associated with improved energy levels, elevated motivation, increased muscle mass, reduced vascular inflammation and decreased fat storage. Body fat contains aromatase, an enzyme that converts testosterone into estrogen. So, if a man carries too much weight in his mid-section his body will produce more estrogens and have reduced testosterone levels. Low testosterone and excess estrogen lead to increased abdominal fat, making this a vicious cycle.

For women, testosterone increases muscle and bone strength, something critical for your exercise and transformation program. Libido, assertiveness and sexual response are also influenced by a woman's testosterone levels.

Optimizing testosterone levels can be a very complex and delicate process, but high-intensity exercise—like metabolic resistance training, (MRT), also known as metabolic strength training—maintaining a healthy weight, L-arginine, zinc, branch chain amino acids, DHA and vitamin D are effective ways to optimize levels.

Dehydroepiandosterone (DHEA) is used as a precursor to the production of male and female sex hormones and is involved in the aging process, cognitive abilities and mood. It aids your transformation by increasing muscle mass, strength and energy levels.

The lesson to be learned from this is there are many more factors other than calories in and calories out that can dramatically influence your body transformation. And exercise is one of the keys to optimize hormone levels to increase your likelihood of success.

CHAPTER 5

Shred Fat, Boost Metabolism and Maximize Lean Muscle Development with Metabolic Resistance Training

Hundreds of thousands of men and women spend hours sweating in the gym to transform their physiques every day. Many of these choose to run on a treadmill, spin the wheels off an exercise bike or pump their legs on an elliptical. However, the overwhelming body of research suggests that a more effective way to shred fat, build lean muscle, boost your metabolism and reveal a physique you can be proud of is through metabolic resistance training (MRT).

MRT is a series, or circuit, of resistance exercises focused on the large muscles of the body performed at high intensity—near maximum effort— with as little rest as possible between sets. The exercises challenge multiple muscles at once—often called compound exercises—and engage the stabilizer muscles that are habitually missed during standard strength training workouts. Quite simply, with MRT you are able to complete more fat-shredding and muscle-building exercises in less time, and maximize your results.

MRT is designed to maximize calorie burn, boost lean muscle mass, while enhancing metabolic rate post workout, which leads to accelerated fat loss. Your metabolic rate is the number of calories you burn while at rest—something that is very important to keep elevated when attempting to manage your weight or transform your body. Research at the Human Performance Center, Anderson University, suggests that explosive metabolic workouts shred calories at a much higher rate when compared to slow or standard exercises. Not only do you burn more calories during your workout—up to nine times more—you get an afterburn effect that leaves your metabolism elevated for up to 72 hours (36-39).

It also revs up and tunes your central nervous system (CNS) and enhances muscle endurance. The stress placed on the CNS is directly proportional to how hard you are training and the weight being used. Since the CNS is involved in athletic performance, muscle endurance, muscle contraction, muscle coordination and strength, it is important to challenge the CNS so that it partners with you to achieve your body transformation.

We just finished discussing how optimized hormones can aid your body transformation, and how exercise influences hormone optimization. Hormones, particularly those associated with fat loss, respond well to MRT, improving your hormone profile. MRT influences the production and release of human growth hormone, epinephrine, testosterone, insulin-like growth factor-1 (IGF-1) and cortisol (40, 41).

Traditional isolation resistance exercises don't challenge your body enough to improve your hormone profile and, in fact, can be damaging to soft tissues. To see results, you need to challenge multiple muscles simultaneously, alternating exercises frequently and progressively increasing the load or weight you use. Your muscles will only give what is asked of them, so repeating the same weight and exercise over and over will not produce sustainable results. You will eventually plateau and stop seeing results. A program designed to alternate exercises and progressively increase loads will produce more rapid and sustainable results, reducing the likelihood that you will plateau.

Lastly, sleep is critical to your overall well-being and particularly important for recovery and weight management. During sleep your body focuses on recovery and muscle growth. The pituitary gland stimulates the production of HGH and protein synthesis occurs, as long as sufficient protein is consumed in the diet. Inadequate sleep influences brain and hormonal activity, which makes you crave high-calorie junk foods, resulting in weight gain. Get a minimum of seven to eight hours of continuous sleep each night, preferably at consistent times.

The evidence is clear that MRT is far more effective for those who want to transform their body rapidly, while successfully sustaining the results.

Maximizing Your Workout
- Focus on the quality of the exercise being performed, doing as many quality reps as you can. Speed can cause injuries if your form is not correct. Follow the old adage "quality over quantity."
- The best time of day to work out is the time when you will always do it. Make daily physical activity a way of life and a habit. Research is

mixed, but there are some valid arguments for morning being the best time to work out.

1. **Melt fat all day.** Carbohydrate reserves are significantly reduced during the long fast of sleeping, causing your body to rely on fat reserves for fuel during your morning workout. In this state, you will shred more fat, when compared to the afternoon and evening when your carbohydrate reserves are full. Even better, because you are employing metabolic resistance training, you will be burning more calories all throughout the day.

2. **Convenience and motivation.** While this isn't true for everyone, mornings usually have less distractions and commitments to prevent you from working out. By working out in the morning you are also prioritizing your health and well-being, making time for you to experience your body transformation. In addition, many people find it difficult to work out in the evening after a hard day at work or long day of caring for their children.

3. **Consistency.** The reality is that about fifty percent of people who begin an exercise program have abandoned it three to six months later. Research suggests that people who work out in the morning are far more likely to stick to it than those who work out in the evenings.

4. **Improved mood**. Exercising produces "feel good" hormones that balance your mood and also decreases the negative effects of stress making you feel better. Starting the day off right with an increase in feel good hormones may improve your entire day.

5. **Optimized testosterone levels**. Testosterone is critical for muscle growth and strength in both men and women. And testosterone levels are typically highest in the morning in both men and women, steadily declining throughout the day.

- For your body transformation to take place, your diet has to be clean as was described in chapter 1. In fact, those sexy abs that we all crave are more about diet than they are endless amounts of crunches. However, in today's world, your body is constantly assaulted by environmental toxins, chemicals and excess stress, leading to less than optimal levels of nutrients to fuel your body. To combat this effect a multi-nutrient is a must. Take a whole food multi-nutrient—to maximize absorption and bioactivity—in divided doses daily.

- The typical American diet contains too many omega-6 fats and too few omega-3 fats. Taking a molecularly distilled marine oil supplement with sufficient antioxidants to preserve the delicate oils is wise for anyone seeking better health or to maintain their current level of health.

- Maintaining hydration is important for exercise performance and overall well-being. Aim to drink four to eight ounces every 10 to 15 minutes during exercise, and rehydrate with approximately 16 to 20 ounces of water after your workout. Some experts suggest weighing before and after exercise, and drinking 16 to 20 ounces per pound lost during your workout.
- One study found that men who added the equivalent of one drop of peppermint essential oil to 500ml of water improved overall exercise performance (42). The study authors concluded that relaxation of bronchial smooth muscles, increases in brain oxygenation and decreases in blood lactate levels were the most likely explanation for the increase in exercise performance.
- Working out with a partner can add a motivational edge to maintain consistency and push yourself harder. In fact, research suggests that working out with a more capable partner can increase your motivation to exercise by as much as 100 percent (43). Plus it's more fun anyway.
- Replenishing electrolytes during exercise is very important to avoid cramps, muscle spasms and an irregular heartbeat. Coconut water is a great natural electrolyte source, whereas "sports drinks" tend to be loaded with sugar, artificial sweeteners or other harmful chemicals.
- Exercise to upbeat, high-tempo music. You may find that your reps are following the beat of your music, so the right music playlist is important to maximize your workout.
- Keep a towel handy to wipe sweat off of your body, especially between circuits.

Recovery
- What you eat post workout can significantly influence your body transformation. Your muscles use glucose and glycogen—stored energy—to fuel your workout. If these levels get severely depleted your body will release cortisol, which signals your body to break down muscle and convert it to glucose for fuel. This is not an optimal situation because it results in muscle loss. Your post-workout meal can prevent this. It is critical to get protein and carbohydrates to the muscles as soon as possible after your workout. Both protein and carbs stimulate muscle growth and encourage muscle recovery. Whey protein is a fast digesting protein and great post workout. The National Strength and Conditioning Association recommends active

people and strength trainers consume 0.4-0.6 grams of protein per pound of body weight. Twenty to 25 grams within 30 minutes of your workout is strongly recommended.

- Athletes and those participating in strenuous exercise will naturally produce more free radicals, making it necessary to provide your body a constant stream of antioxidants from both diet and supplementation. Superfruit health beverages contain significant quantities of antioxidants and other beneficial nutrients, making them a great choice to reduce oxidative stress from free radicals. One word of caution, some muscle damage is necessary in order to strengthen and enlarge your muscles, so don't go to extreme's with antioxidants.

- As your body adapts to a different exercise routine and you constantly change the way you challenge your muscles throughout the TransformWise training system, you are bound to experience some muscle soreness. The best thing you can do is rub your major muscles with a pain relieving ointment—like essential oils or arnica—immediately following your post-exercise shower. This will reduce muscle soreness and aid the recovery process so you are ready for the next day's workout.

Protection

- Some individuals need added protection for their muscles, soft tissues, bones and joints. If you want to protect these tissues a supplement containing a combination of glucosamine, chondroitin methylsulfonylmethane and other supportive nutrients may be an option worth considering.

- Beyond providing healthy fats, marine oil supplements support joint, heart, brain and eye health, and aid the normal inflammatory response.

CHAPTER 6

The TransformWise Training System

EQUIPMENT

Interval timer (Free apps from Google Play or the App Store or a GymBoss interval timer)

Swiss or stability ball (appropriate for your size)
Height/Ball Size
5' or under/45 cm
5'1" - 5'8"/55 cm
5'9" – 6'2"/65 cm
6'3" – 6'7"/75 cm
6'8" and taller/85 cm

Dumbbell set (rubber coated hex preferred)
Beginner – 3 to 15 lb. set
Intermediate – 5 to 20 lb. set
Advanced – 10 to 35 lb. set

Kettlebell(s)
Beginner – 5 to 15 lb.
Intermediate – 10 to 20 lb.
Advanced – 15 to 35+ lb.

Comfortable clothes

Exercise Mat

Water bottle

Sweat Towel

Music Player

Workout Gloves

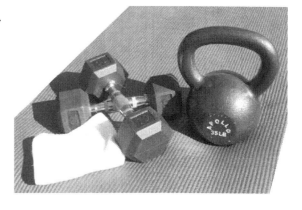

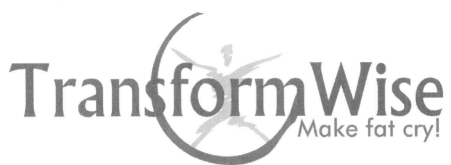

FITNESS TEST

This test is intended to help determine your current fitness level, track results and guide load and duration of exercises. This fitness test should be performed before beginning the program, and again every 4 weeks to track progress. Prior to performing this test it is important that you warm up your muscles. Please follow the pre-workout warm-up routine before beginning the fitness test.

PRE-WORKOUT WARM-UP AND STRETCH

Also perform before each daily workout to reduce injuries and post-exercise soreness and to prepare your body for the increased demands of exercise.

~Jog in place 30-60 seconds
~ Perform 30-60 seconds of jumping jacks
~ Perform 30-60 seconds of arm swings (rotate your arms forward and backward like a windmill)
~ Stretch shoulders, back, upper and lower legs and groin

1 – PUSHUPS (Upper body)

Men should use the standard pushup positions with only your hands and toes touching the floor. Your body should form a straight line from your head to your heels and your head should be looking slightly ahead not straight down. Place your hands slightly wider than shoulder-width apart. Lower your chest down towards the floor until your elbows are at a right angle of your chest is just off the ground. Press up until you are back in the original position and repeat. Women may use the modified pushup position, with knees on the ground following the same procedure as above. Breathe in as you lower and exhale as you push back up.

Do as many pushups as you can until failure and record your score.

Start	Week 4	Week 8	Week 12

Men, based on age	18-29	30-39	40-49	50-59	60+
Beginner	0-24	0-19	0-15	0-10	0-7
Intermediate	25-49	20-44	16-39	11-34	8-29
Advanced	50+	45+	40+	35+	30+
Women (modified), based on age	18-29	30-39	40-49	50-59	60+
Beginner	0-15	0-12	0-9	0-7	0-5
Intermediate	16-39	13-31	10-28	8-25	6-19
Advanced	40+	32+	29+	26+	20+

2 – Jumping Jacks (Cardio, coordination, endurance)

Stand erect with your arms at your side, feet straight and close together, head straight and looking forward. Bend your knees slightly and jump up. While in the air spread your legs out slightly wider than shoulder width apart. Simultaneously raise your arms up over your head until they touch above your head. Quickly jump back to the starting position and repeat the process.

Perform jumping jacks for one minute, counting each full repetition and record your score.

Start	Week 4	Week 8	Week 12

Men & Women, based on age	18-29	30-39	40-49	50-59	60+
Beginner	0-30	0-25	0-20	0-15	0-8
Intermediate	31-60	26-55	21-50	16-39	9-28
Advanced	61+	56+	51+	40+	29+

3 – Wall Squat (Lower body, legs, muscle endurance)

Stand with your head and back against a wall arms hanging at your side. Feet should be shoulder width apart and about 18 inches from the wall. Lower your body into a squat position with your thighs parallel to the floor. Hold this position.

Maintain this position until failure and record the number of seconds you held the wall squat.

Start	Week 4	Week 8	Week 12

Men, based on age	18-29	30-39	40-49	50-59	60+
Beginner	0-35	0-30	0-25	0-20	0-15
Intermediate	36-74	31-64	26-54	21-44	16-39
Advanced	75+	65+	55+	45+	40+
Women, based on age	18-29	30-39	40-49	50-59	60+
Beginner	0-30	0-25	0-20	0-15	0-10
Intermediate	31-59	26-49	21-39	16-34	11-29
Advanced	60+	50+	40+	35+	30+

4 – Forearm Plank (Core, lower back, upper body)

Start in a pushup position except your forearms are on the ground instead of your hands. Ensure your elbows line up directly underneath your shoulders. Form a straight line from you head to your heals—place a broomstick or other straight object on your back to make sure you are in the correct position. Squeeze your glutes and tighten your abdominals. Hold this position.

Maintain this position until failure and record the number of seconds you held the plank.

Start	Week 4	Week 8	Week 12

Men & Women, based on age	18-29	30-39	40-49	50-59	60+
Beginner	0-70	0-65	0-60	0-45	0-35
Intermediate	71-119	66-99	61-89	46-79	36-59
Advanced	120+	100+	90+	80+	60+

5 – Modified Sit and Reach Flexibility Test (Lower back and hamstring flexibility)

Sit on the floor with your feet flat against a wall, and your legs toughing the floor. Reach forward as far as you can with your hands and note how far you are able to reach.

Do this three times and record your best score.

Start	Week 4	Week 8	Week 12

39

Men & Women	All Ages
Beginner	Fingers short of wall
Intermediate	Fingers touch wall
Advanced	Knuckles or palms touch wall

6 – Shoulder Joint Flexibility Test (Shoulder flexibility)

While standing, raise either arm straight above your head. Bend your elbow and reach down across your back with your palm facing your upper back. Position your opposite arm down behind your back and reach up across your back, again with you hand against your back. Keeping your fingers extended, try to overlap the fingers of your upper hand over your lower hand. Repeat with arms reversed, so the arm that was on top is now in the bottom position.

Do this three times and record your best score.

Start	Week 4	Week 8	Week 12

Men & Women	All Ages
Beginner	Fingers don't touch
Intermediate	Fingers touch
Advanced	Fingers overlap

Cool Down and Stretch

Also perform after each daily workout.

~ Walk in place for two minutes
~ Stretch shoulders, back, upper and lower legs and groin

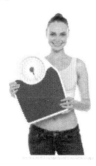

Measurements/Tracking

How to measure	Before	Week 4	Week 8	Week 12
Weight Weigh yourself on a scale and record your weight. Don't let this discourage you. If you are training properly you may be adding muscle, which makes the scale refuse to budge.				
Body Fat % Have your body fat measured by a professional, purchase skin calipers to measure body fat at home, or use a special scale designed to measure body composition.				
Waist Place the tape measure about ½ inch below your belly button, or wherever your waist is smallest. Exhale and measure your torso before inhaling again.				
Hips Place the tape measure across the widest part of your hips/buttocks and measure all the way around.				
Right Bicep Wrap the tape measure around the highest peak or largest area of your right bicep and measure all the way around.				
Left Bicep Wrap the tape measure around the highest peak or largest area of your left bicep and measure all the way around.				
Right Thigh Wrap the tape measure around the same spot on your right thigh each time and measure all the way around.				
Left Thigh Wrap the tape measure around the same spot on your left thigh each time and measure all the way around.				
Bust/Chest Lift up your arms, wrap the tape measure around your chest at nipple level for women or just above the nipple for men, then lower your arms and measure all the way around.				
Pictures May be the most important measure! Stand in front of a mirror and take a picture of yourself in a bathing suit, shorts and sports bra, or just shorts for the men. Take another picture of your profile view. Or recruit someone to take photos. Take pictures weekly if so desired.				
Clothes Lastly, the way your clothes fit is an excellent measure of your body transformation. If they are fitting looser, chances are you have lost inches. If your shirts have a hard time accommodating your bulging biceps and chest, you have added lean muscle.				

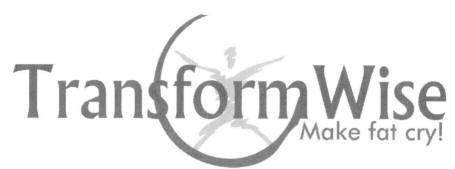

WORKOUT SCHEDULE

Choose a workout track (beginner, intermediate or advanced) based on your overall fitness test results, current state of health and fitness goals.

Beginners perform all 10 exercises for 30 seconds each at or near maximum ability followed by 15 seconds of rest between each exercise to complete one circuit. Complete 2 circuits, with 2 minutes rest between circuits. Increase to Intermediate level workout after week 2 and increase to Advanced level workout after week 4.

Intermediate perform all 10 exercises for 45 seconds each at or near maximum ability followed by 15 seconds of rest between each exercise to complete one circuit. Complete 3 circuits, with 2 minutes rest between circuits. Increase to Advanced level workout after week 2.

Advanced perform all 10 exercises for 60 seconds each at or near maximum ability followed by 15 seconds of rest after each exercise to complete one circuit. Complete 3 circuits, with 2 minutes rest between circuits.

Each group should work to progressively increase the load (weight) and number of reps completed in each circuit. And leave everything on the mat during your third round of each workout. Make this you're your best and empty your tank—you'll have time to recover before your next fat-shredding workout. Modified Versions of the exercise are listed in parentheses when available. If you need to rest for a few seconds during an exercise this is okay. When you are just starting some people find it beneficial to perform difficult exercises in sets of five or 10.

Free days are intended for you to choose any physical activity you enjoy. This can be any form of exercise, yoga, participate in a sport, walking, rollerblading, or just about anything else that provides 30 to 60 minutes of physical activity.

Flexibility has been built in to your workout schedule so you can find a track that works best for you. Choose your favorite workout or physical activity on free days. Participating in cardio high-intensity interval training for two of the free days each week will accelerate your body transformation.

Upon completion of the 12-week exercise program, you may start from the beginning following the same workout schedule or create your own custom routine based on the 12 workouts.

*** For printable PDF copies of the fitness test, measurements and workouts go to http://goo.gl/kHz6Qc and enter the code IWILLTRANSFORM ***

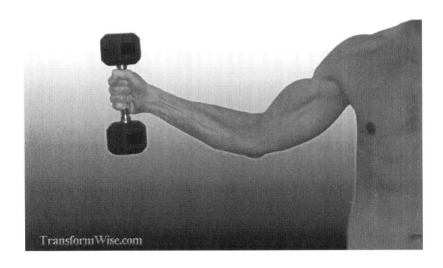

Scott A. Johnson

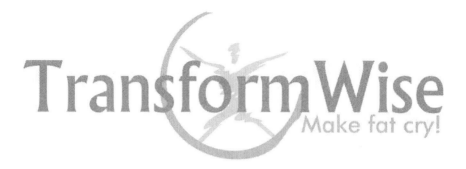

WORKOUT SCHEDULE

FOUNDATION

	Day 1	Day 2	Day 3	Day 4	Day 5	Day 6	Day 7
Week 1	#1	Free	#2	Free	#1	Free/Rest	Rest
Week 2	#2	Free	#1	Free	#2	Free/Rest	Rest

CONDITIONING

	Day 1	Day 2	Day 3	Day 4	Day 5	Day 6	Day 7
Week 3	#3	Free	#4	Free	#3	Free/Rest	Rest
Week 4	#4	Free	#3	Free	#4	Free/Rest	Rest

TRANSFORMATION

	Day 1	Day 2	Day 3	Day 4	Day 5	Day 6	Day 7
Week 5	#5	Free	#6	Free	#5	Free/Rest	Rest
Week 6	#6	Free	#5	Free	#6	Free/Rest	Rest
Week 7	#7	Free	#8	Free	#7	Free/Rest	Rest
Week 8	#8	Free	#7	Free	#8	Free/Rest	Rest
Week 9	#9	Free	#10	Free	#9	Free/Rest	Rest
Week 10	#10	Free	#9	Free	#10	Free/Rest	Rest
Week 11	#11	Free	#12	Free	#11	Free/Rest	Rest
Week 12	#12	Free	#11	Free	#12	Free/Rest	Rest

PRE-WORKOUT WARM-UP AND STRETCH

Perform before each daily workout to reduce injuries and post-exercise soreness and to prepare your body for the increased demands of exercise.
~ Jog in place 30-60 seconds
~ Perform 30-60 seconds of jumping jacks
~ Perform 30-60 seconds of arm swings (each arm)
~ Stretch shoulders, back, upper and lower legs and groin

COOL DOWN AND STRETCH

Also perform after each daily workout.
~ Walk in place or short circles for two minutes
~ Stretch shoulders, back, upper and lower legs and groin

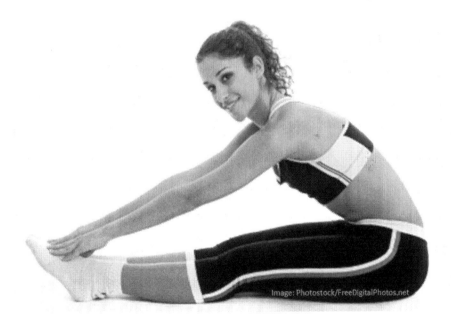

Image: Photostock/FreeDigitalPhotos.net

For examples of the exercises in each workout visit:
http://www.youtube.com/user/sjohnson2221/videos

Scott A. Johnson

WORKOUT #1

1 - Kettlebell Swings (Dumbbell Swings)
2 - Pushups (Modified Pushup)
3 - Dumbbell Thrusters (Prisoner Squats)
4 - Bicycle Crunches (Raised Leg Crunches)
5 - Alternating Front Lunge (No Modified)
6 - Stability Ball Double Dumbbell Press (Single Dumbbell Floor Press)
7 - Plank Abduction (Plank on Knees)
8 - Kettlebell/Dumbbell Goblet Squats (Crossed Arm Squats)
9 - Jumping Jacks (Modified Jumping Jacks, One Leg at a time)
10 - Oblique Twists on Stability Ball (Oblique Twists)

WORKOUT #2

1 - Kettlebell Side Swings (Dumbbell Side Swings)
2 - Pike Pushups (Modified Pushups)
3 - Sprawls (Half Sprawls)
4 - Russian Twist with Dumbbell (Russian Twist with Legs on Floor)
5 - Reverse Lunge (No Modified)
6 - Double Dumbbell Clean and Press (Single Dumbbell Clean and Press)
7 - Stability Ball Crunches (No Modified)
8 - Squat with Front Kick (Squat with Side Leg Raise)
9 - High Knees (Knee to Hand Raise)
10 - Glute Bridge (No Modified)

WORKOUT #3

1 - Kettlebell Leg Pass Through (No Modified)

2 - Stability Ball Incline Pushups (Modified Pushups)

3 - Burpees no Pushup (Burpees to Knee Pushup Position and Stand up)

4 -Single Leg V-ups (Single Leg V-ups With Back on Ground)

5 - Ski Jump Squats (Hindu Squats)

6 - Alternating Dumbbell Shoulder Press (Single Dumbbell Shoulder Press)

7 - Plank to Pushup (Plank to Pushup on Knees)

8 - Crossback Lunge (Crossback Lunge not as deep)

9 - Mountain Climbers (Plank with Alternate Knee to Chest)

10 - Pointer Dog (No Modified)

WORKOUT #4

1 - Two Arm Kettlebell Swings with High Pulls (No Modified)

2 - Pushup Jacks (Modified Pushups)

3 - Sprinter Pulls (Alternate High Knee Raises)

4 - Spread Eagle Sit Ups (Sit Ups)

5 - Double Dumbbell Squat and Press (Single Dumbbell Squat and Press)

6 - Stability Ball Dumbbell Fly (No Modified)

7 - Stability Ball Leg Curls (Stability Ball Leg Curls Back Completely on Floor)

8 - Warrior Side Lunge (Warrior Forward Lunge)

9 - Wide Leg Runs (Wide Leg Knee Raises)

10 - Plank Single Leg Raise (Plank or Plank on Knees)

WORKOUT #5

1 - Alternate Single Arm Kettlebell Swings (Kettlebell Swings)
2 - Swoop Pushups (Modified Pushups)
3 - Reverse Burpees (No Modified)
4 - Threading the Needle Side Planks (Side Plank)
5 - Squat with Knee Raise (Prisoner Squat)
6 - Stability Ball Dumbbell Press (Stability Ball Single Dumbbell Press)
7 - Plank Jacks (Plank Single Alternating Leg Spread Out)
8 - Saddlebag Slimmers (No Modified)
9 - Tadpole to Frog (Tadpole to Frog, Walking Legs up to Arms)
10 - Marching on Stability Ball Glute Bridge (No Modified)

WORKOUT #6

1 - Alternating Single Arm Kettlebell Overhead Swing (Kettlebell Swings)
2 - Pushups Single Leg Raise (Modified Pushups)
3 - Alternating Kettlebell Diagonal Lift (Alternating Diagonal Lift without Kettlebell)
4 - Abs in and Outs (Knee to Chest then Extend Legs)
5 - Frog Squat (Frog Squat with Hands on Floor)
6 - Stability Ball Triceps Dips (Tricep Dips without Stability Ball)
7 - Stability Ball Plank (Plank)
8 - Alternating Pulse Lunges (Alternating Front Lunges)
9 - Toe Taps on a Kettlebell (No Modified)
10 - Superman/woman over Stability Ball (Modified Superman/woman Over Stability Ball, Arms Behind)

WORKOUT #7

1 - Kettlebell Squat and Upright Row (Goblet Squat)
2 - Diamond Pushups (Modified Diamond Pushups on Knees)
3 - Rotating Sprawl (Plank Side to Side Hop)
4 - Stability Ball Leg Raises (Leg Raises)
5 - Standing Calf Raises (No modified)
6 - Double Dumbbell Deadlift and Curl (Single Dumbbell Two-hand Grip Deadlift and Curl)
7 - Pike Roll Out on Stability Ball (Pike to Plank)
8 - Reverse Lunge and Knee Raise (Reverse Lunge)
9 - Run Around Kettlebell (No Modified)
10 - Table Makers (No Modified)

WORKOUT #8

1 - Walking Forward and Backward Kettlebell Swings (Kettlebell Swings)
2 - Pushup Knee to Elbow (Modified Pushup Knee to Elbow)
3 - Alternating Side Leg Circles (No modified)
4 - V-ups (Modified V-ups With Back on Ground)
5 - Squat to Alternating Front to Rear Lunge (Squat-Front Lungs-Squat-Rear Lunge)
6 - Cross Body Single Arm Dumbbell Clean and Press (Cross Body Two Hand Dumbbell Clean and Press)
7 - Stability Ball Knee Tucks (Plank to Pike)
8 - Alternating Glute Activation Lunges (Forward Lunge)
9 - Speed Skaters (Lateral Step Back Side to Side)
10 - Flutter Kicks (No Modified)

Scott A. Johnson

WORKOUT #9

1 - Wide Leg Double Dumbbell Deadlift and Upright Row (Single Dumbbell Deadlift and Upright Row)
2 - Pushup with Alternating Renegade Rows (Modified Pushups with Renegade Rows)
3 - Donkey Kicks (Table with Alternating Front Kicks)
4 - Abs Spring Ups (Legs Straight Abs Spring Ups)
5 - Kettlebell Weighted Standing Calf Raises (Standing Calf Raises)
6 - Kettlebell Pullovers (Kettlebell Press)
7 - Stability Ball Alternating Oblique Crunches (Oblique Crunches)
8 - Alternate Side Lunge with Dumbbell Press Out (Alternate Side Lunge)
9 - Up and Out Jacks (Modified Jumping Jacks, One Leg at a Time)
10 - Shoulder Bridge with One Leg Raised (Glute Bridge)

WORKOUT #10

1 - Man Makers (Burpee with Pushup)
2 - T Pushups (Modified Pushups With Single Arm Raise)
3 - Mountain Climber Sprawls (Mountain Climbers)
4 - Plank Knee to Elbow (Plank)
5 - Inverted Flyers (Posterior Leg Raises on Hands and Knees)
6 - Dumbbell Bent Over Rows (Single Dumbbell Both Hands Grip Bent Over Row)
7 - Windshield Wipers (Russian Twist)
8 - Alternating Front Lunge with Twist (Front Lunge)
9 - High Kicks (No Modified)
10 - Reverse plank (No Modified)

WORKOUT #11

1 - Inchworms Forward and Back (No Modified)

2 - Stability Ball Pushups (Modified Pushups or Midsection on Ball Pushups)

3 - Renegade Rows (Modified Pushup Position Renegade Rows)

4 - Bicycle Crunches (Raised Leg Crunches)

5 - Squat to Side Warrior Lunge (Deep Squats)

6 - Kettlebell Pass-Pass-Pass-Press (Pass-Pass-Pass-Press without Kettlebell)

7 - Stability Ball Ab Pass (Back on Floor and Pass Ball Back and Forth)

8 - Side Lunge with Floor Touch (Warrior Side Lunge)

9 - Alternate Rear Kicks (No Modified)

10 - Side Plank with Oblique Crunch (Oblique Crunch)

WORKOUT #12

1 - Push Jerks with Kettlebell (Push Jerks, No Weights)

2 - Negative Pushups on Dumbbells (Modified Pushups)

3 - Weighted Standing Calf Raises (Standing Calf Raises)

4 - Stability Ball Roll Outs (No modified)

5 - Front to Rear Lunges (Front or Rear Lunges)

6 - Dive Bombers (Modified Pushups Position Dive Bombers)

7 - Heal Touch (No Modified)

8 - Figure Eight Flutter Kicks (Figure Eight Flutter Kicks Smaller Circles)

9 - Lateral hops (Side to Side Shuffles)

10 - Stability Ball Alternate Shoulder Press (Standing Alternate Shoulder Press)

###

Once you have completed the program, you will want to show off your new physique and display your new found strength with a TransformWise t-shirt. You are now part of a very select group and deserve recognition for it. Purchase yours at http://goo.gl/pkxPvy today and wear it with pride.

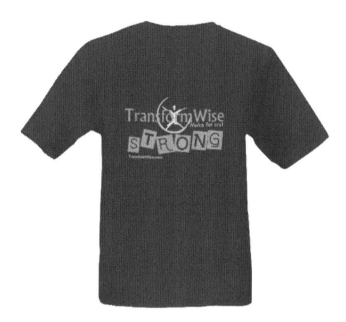

About the Author:

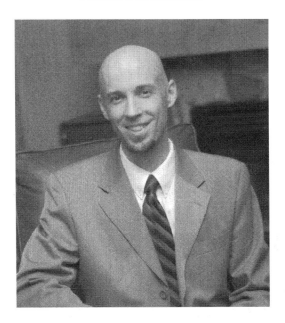

Scott Johnson is the author of four books and more than 250 articles featured in online and print publications and is considered an expert on health, fitness and nutraceuticals. He has a doctorate in naturopathy and is a board certified Alternative Medical Practitioner (AMP). Scott draws on his wealth of experience and diverse educational background to share the secrets of natural healing with those who seek greater wellness.

Connect with Scott:

FACEBOOK: https://www.facebook.com/author.scott.johnson
TWITTER: https://twitter.com/DocScottJohnson

Scott A. Johnson

REFERENCES

(1) Arnold LM, Ball MJ, Mann J. Effect of isoenergetic intake of three to nine meals on plasma lipoproteins and glucose metabolism. *Am J Clin Nutr.* 1993 Mar;57(3):446-51.
(2) Jenkins D, et al. Nibbling versus gorging: Metabolic advantages of increasing meal frequency. *N Engl J Med.* 1989 Oct 5;321(14):929-34.
(3) Edelstein SL, et al. Increased meal frequency associated with decreased cholesterol concentrations; Rancho Bernardo, CA, 1984-1987. *Am J Clin Nutr.* 1992 Mar;55(3):664-9.
(4) Farshchi HR, Taylor MA, Macdonald IA. Beneficial metabolic effects of regular meal frequency on dietary thermogenesis, insulin sensitivity, and fasting lipid profiles in healthy obese women. *Am J Clin Nutr.* 2005 Jan;81(1):16-24.
(5) Toschke AM, et al. Meal frequency and childhood obesity. *Obes Res.* 2005 Nov;13(11):1932-8.
(6) Jääskeläinen A, et al. Associations of meal frequency and breakfast with obesity and metabolic syndrome traits in adolescents of Northern Finland Birth Cohort 1986. *Nutr Metab Cardiovasc Dis.* 2012 Aug 14. [Epub ahead of print]
(7) Speechly DP, Buffenstein R. Greater appetite control associated with an increased frequency of eating in lean males. *Appetite.* 1999 Dec;33(3):285-97.
(8) Ceriello A. Postprandial Hyperglycemia and Cardiovascular Disease. *Endocri Pract.* 2006 Jan-Feb;12 Suppl 1:47-51.
(9) Fava S. Role of postprandial hyperglycemia in cardiovascular disease. *Expert Rev Cardiovasc Ther.* 2008 Jul;6(6):859-72. doi: 10.1586/14779072.6.6.859.
(10)   Arnold L, Ball M, Duncan A, Mann J. Effect of isoenergetic intake of three or nine meals on plasma lipoproteins and glucose metabolism. *AM J Clin Nutr.* 1993 Mar;57(3):446-51.
(11)   Jenkins D, Wolever T, Vuksan V, et al. Nibbling versus gorging: Metabolic advantages of increased meal frequency. *N Engl J Med.* 1989 Oct;321:929-934.
(12)   Edelstein S, Barrett-Connor EL, Wingard DL, Cohn BA. Increased meal frequency associated with decreased cholesterol concentrations; Rancho Bernardo, CA, 1984-1987. *Am J Clin Nutr.* 1992 Mar;55(3):664-9.

(13)   Toschke A, Kuchenhoff H, Koletzko B, von Kries R. Meal frequency and childhood obesity. *Obes Res.* 2005;13(11):1932-8.

(14)   Farshchi H, Taylor M, Macdonald I. Beneficial metabolic effects of regular meal frequency on dietary thermogenesis, insulin sensitivity, and fasting lipid profiles in healthy obese women. *Am J Clin Nutr.* 2005 Jan;81(1):16-24.

(15)   LeBlanc J, Mercier I, Nadeau A. Components of postprandial thermogenesis in relation to meal frequency in humans. *Can J Physiol Pharmacol.* 1993 Dec;71(12):879-83.

(16)   Arciero P, Simon, J Ruby M, Clippinger B, Gerson L. Increased dietary protein and meal frequency improves postprandial thermogenesis in obese men and women. *FASEBJ.* 2007;21:111.2.

(17)   Speechly D, Buffenstein R. Greater appetite control associated with an increased frequency of eating in lean males. *Appetite.* 1999 Dec;33(3):285-97.

(18)   La Bounty P, Campbell B, Wilson J, et al. International society of sports nutrition position stand: meal frequency. *J Int Soc Sports Nutr.* 2011 Mar 16;8:4.

(19)   Speechly D, Rogers G, Buffenstein R. Acute appetite reduction associated with an increased frequency of eating in obese males. *Int J Obes Relat Metab Disord.* 1999 Nov;23(11):1151-9.

(20)   Vatansever-Ozen S, Tiryaki-Sonmez G, Bugdayci G, Ozen G. The effects of exercise on food intake and hunger: Relationship with acylated ghrelin and leptin. *J of Sports Sci and Med.* 2011;10:283-91.

(21)   Flores M, Fernandez M, Ropelle E, et al. Exercise improves insulin and leptin sensitivity in hypothalamus of Wistar rats. *Diabetes.* 2006 Sep;55(9):2554-61.

(22)   Kang S, Kim K, Shin K. Exercise training improves leptin sensitivity in peripheral tissue of obese rats. *Biochem Biophys Res Commun.* 2013 Jun 7;435(#):454-9.

(23)   Ropelle E, Flores M, Cintra D, et al. IL-6 and IL-10 Anti-Inflammatory Activity Links Exercise to Hypothalamic Insulin and Leptin Sensitivity through IKKb and ER Stress Inhibition. *PLoS Biol.* 2010 Aug 24;8(8).

(24)   Saunders T, Palombella A, McGuire A, et al. Acute exercise increases adiponectin levels in abdominally obese men. *J Nutr Metab.* 2012;2012:148729.

(25)   Kriketos A, Gan S, Poynten A, Furler S, Chrisholm D, Campbell L. Exercise increases adiponectin levels and insulin sensitivity in humans. *Diabetes Care.* 2004 Feb;27(2):629-30.
(26)   Belalcazar L, Lang W, Haffer S. Adiponectin and the mediation of HDL-cholesterol change with improved lifestyle: the Look AHEAD Study. *J Lipid Res.* 2012 Dec;53(12):2726-33.
(27)   WU J, Cahill L, Mozaffarian. Effect of fish oil on circulating adiponectin: A systematic review and meta-analysis of randomized controlled trials. *J Clin Endocrinol Metab.* 2013 Jun;98(6):2451-9.
(28)   Houmard J, Tanner C, Slentz C, Duscha B, McCartney J, Kraus W. Effect of the volume and intensity of exercise training on insulin sensitivity. *J Appl Physiol.*2004 Jan;96(1):101-6.
(29)   Van Proeyen K, Szlufcik K, Nielens H, et al. Training in the fasted state improves glucose tolerance during fat-rich diet. *J Physiol.* 2010 Nov 1;588(Pt 21):4289-302.
(30)   Thomas G, Kraemer W, Comstock B, Dunn-Lewis Cm Maresh C, Volek J. Obesity, growth hormone and exercise. *Sports Med.* 2013 Sep;43(9):839-49.
(31)   Wideman L, Weltman J, Hartman M, Veldhuis J, Weltman A. Growth hormone release during acute and chronic aerobic and resistance exercise: recent findings. *Sports Med.* 2002;32(15):987-1004.
(32)   Felsig N, Brasel J, Cooper D. Effect of low and high intesntiy exercise on circulating growth hormone. *J Clin Endocrinol Metab.* 1992 Jul;75(1):157-62.
(33)   Cappon J, Brasel J, Mohan S, Cooper D. Effect of brief exercise on circulating insulin-like growth factor. *J Appl Physiol.* 1994 Jun;76(6):2490-6.
(34)   Mackie A, Rafiee H, Malcom P, Salt L, van Aken G. Specific food structures suppress appetite through reduced gastric emptying rate. *Am J Physiol Gastrointest Liver Physiol.* 2013 Jun 1;304(11):G1038-43.
(35)   McHugh P, Moran T. The stomach, cholecystokinin, and satiety. *Fed Proc.* 1986 Apr;45(5):1384-90.
(36)   Perry C, Heigenhauser G, Bonen A, Sprite L. High-intensity aerobic interval training increases fat and carbohydrate metabolic capcities in human skeletal muscle. *Appl Physiol Nutr Metab.* 2008 Dec;33(6):1112-23.
(37)   Tesch P, Colliander E, Kaiser P. Muscle metabolism during intense, heavy-resistance exercise. *Eur J Appl Physiol Occup Physiol.* 1986;55(4):362-6.

(38)   Heden T, Lox C, Rose P, Reid S, Kirk E. One-set resistance training elevates energy expenditure for 72 h similar to three sets. *Eur J Appl Physiol.* 2011 Mar;111(3):477-84.

(39)   Hackney K, Engels H, Gretebeck R. Resting energy expenditure and delayed-onset muscle soreness after full-body resistance training with an eccentric concentration. *J Strength Cond Res.* 2008 Sep;22(5):1602-9.

(40)   Kraemer W, Ratamess N. Hormonal responses and adaptations to resistance exercise training. *Sports Med.* 2005;35(4):339-61.

(41)   Kraemer W, Hakkinen K, Newton R, et al. Effects of heavy-resistance training on hormonal response patterns in younger vs. older men. *J Appl Physiol.* 1999 Sep;87(3):982-92.

(42)   Meamarbashi A, Rajabi A. The effects of peppermint on exercise performance. *J Int Soc Sports Nutr.* 2013 Mar 21;10(1):15.

(43)   Pedersen T. Exercising with a partner boosts motivation. *Psych Central.* 2012. Retrieved September 30, 2013 from http://psychcentral.com/news/2012/05/30/exercising-with-a-partner-boosts-motivation/39421.html.

Scott A. Johnson

RECIPES

Berry Spinach Smoothie
Serves 2

4 to 8 oz. of plain or vanilla almond milk
Two large handfuls of spinach or kale
Two cupped hands worth of berries
Two large spoonfuls of plain or honey Greek yogurt
One large banana
Two servings of protein powder

Directions:
Add all ingredients to blender and blend until smooth. Enjoy.

Nut Butter Spinach Smoothie
Serves 2

4 to 8 oz. of plain or vanilla almond milk
Two large handfuls of spinach or kale
Two large spoonfuls of almond or peanut butter
Two large spoonfuls of plain or honey Greek yogurt
One large banana
Two servings of chocolate protein powder

Directions:
Add all ingredients to blender and blend until smooth. Enjoy.

Oatmeal Blueberry Pancakes
Serves 4 to 6 generously

1 1/2 cups rolled oats
1/2 cup whole-wheat or almond flour
1 tablespoon honey
1/4 teaspoon sea salt
1 teaspoon baking soda
1 1/2 teaspoons baking powder
4 tablespoons olive oil
2 eggs
2 cups buttermilk
1 cup fresh blueberries

Directions:
Lightly oil griddle with olive or coconut oil and heat over medium heat. In large bowl, beat eggs. Mix in all other ingredients, except blueberries, until smooth. Fold in blueberries. Pour or spoon approximately 1/4 cup batter onto griddle for each pancake. Brown both sides and serve warm with Yacon or pure maple syrup.

Whole-grain Peanut Butter and Banana Waffles
Serves 4 to 6 generously

1 cup rolled oats
1 cup whole-wheat or almond flour
1 tablespoon honey
1/4 teaspoon sea salt
1 teaspoon baking soda
1 1/2 teaspoons baking powder
1 ripe banana mashed
1/2 cup peanut or almond butter
2 tablespoons olive oil
2 eggs
2 cups buttermilk
1 teaspoon pure vanilla

Directions:
Beat eggs in large mixing bowl. Mix in all other ingredients until smooth. Cook waffles according to your waffle iron's directions. Serve warm and top with banana slices and Yacon or pure maple syrup.

Spinach Salad with Grilled Chicken, Raspberries and Pecans
Serves 2

Dressing:
6 – 8 fresh or frozen raspberries
1 tablespoon balsamic vinegar
1/2 teaspoon dry Dijon mustard
1 1/2 teaspoons minced, peeled fresh ginger
1 garlic clove, minced and mashed
1/4 teaspoon black pepper
1/2 cup olive oil
1/2 teaspoon poppy seeds

Scott A. Johnson

Blend all ingredients in a blender and store in refrigerator to let flavors meld.

Chicken Breast:
1 whole skinless chicken breast
1 tablespoon grated lemon zest
1/4 cup finely chopped oregano (or 1 tablespoon dried)
2 tablespoons olive oil
1/4 teaspoon black pepper
Juice from one freshly squeezed lemon
2 cupped hands of raspberries
Two thumb sized servings of chopped pecans.

Make marinade in a small bowl by whisking together lemon zest, oregano, olive oil, black pepper and lemon juice. Place chicken breast in zip lock bag with marinade and shake to coat. Let marinate at room temperature for 30 minutes turning bag occasionally.

Cook chicken on grill over medium heat until well browned and cooked through. Cut chicken into 1/4 inch thick slices.

Place large handful of spinach on plate. Cover with desired amount of dressing. Add half of the chicken slices and top with fresh raspberries. Add pecans if desired. Repeat for second serving.

Baked Salmon Salad with Grapefruit, Avocados and Pistachios
Serves 6 – Salmon Recipe Courtesy Gailann Greene

1 (2 to 2 1/2-pound) salmon fillet
1/4 cup olive oil
1 lemon
1/4 teaspoon sea salt
1/4 teaspoon cracked Szechwan pepper
1/2 cup fresh dill

3 handfuls of spinach
3 handfuls of mixed greens
2 Ruby Red Grapefruits
2 cupped hands of pistachio nuts, shelled
2 avocados
Balsamic Vinaigrette

Directions:
Preheat oven to 400 degrees Fahrenheit. Place a sheet of parchment paper on the bottom of a roasting pan and drizzle paper with olive oil. Place salmon on the paper skin side down and drizzle with olive oil, followed by a squeeze of fresh lemon, sea salt, Szechwan pepper and dill. Bake until done, salmon will be flaky (approximately 12-15 minutes). Place salmon on top of serving of mixed greens and top with a serving of grapefruit wedges (peeled and cut into chunks), pistachios, avocado slices and Balsamic vinaigrette.

Mixed berries, Pecan, Tomato and Pan-seared Chicken Breast Salad
Serves 2

1 handful spinach
1 handful mixed greens
2 cupped hands of mixed berries
1 cupped hand of chopped pecans
1 cupped hand cherry tomatoes
1 skinless chicken breast
2 tablespoons olive oil
1/4 teaspoon sea salt
1/4 teaspoon black pepper
1 teaspoon fresh rosemary
2 sprigs fresh thyme
1 garlic cloves minced
Vinegar and olive oil for dressing

Directions:
Heat a skillet over medium high heat. Drizzle half of the olive oil on the chicken breast and add salt and pepper. Put chicken in skillet upside down and add garlic, thyme, rosemary and the rest of the olive oil. When the chicken is golden brown turn over and cook until both sides are well browned and chicken is cooked through. Slice chicken into 1/4 inch thick pieces. Toss spinach and mixed greens in large bowl. Add berries, pecans, tomatoes, olive oil and vinegar to taste. Toss until mixed. Add chicken and serve.

Turkey, Cranberry Swiss Cheese Panini
Serves 1

2 slices wholemeal or sprouted grain Panini bread
Palm sized slice of turkey breast
1 slice of swiss cheese
3/4 teaspoon mustard paste
1/4 cup cranberry sauce
1/4 cup sprouts

Handful of mixed vegetables
Hummus

Directions:
Place mustard paste on one slice of Panini bread with cranberry sauce on the other slice. Add turkey, cheese and sprouts. Toast in toaster until cheese is melted and bread is toasted brown. Serve with steamed mixed vegetables and hummus.

Pan-seared Chicken Breast with Brown Rice, Mixed Vegetables and Hummus
Serves 2

1 skinless chicken breast
2 tablespoons olive oil
1/4 teaspoon sea salt
1/4 teaspoon black pepper
1 teaspoon fresh rosemary
2 sprigs fresh thyme
1 garlic cloves minced

Two cupped hands of brown rice
Two handfuls mixed vegetables
Hummus

Directions:
Cook rice according to package or rice cooker directions. Heat a skillet over medium high heat. Drizzle half of the olive oil on the chicken breast and add salt and pepper. Put chicken in skillet upside down and add garlic, thyme, rosemary and the rest of the olive oil. When the chicken is golden brown turn over and cook until both sides are well browned and chicken is cooked through. Enjoy warm over brown rice with steamed vegetables an hummus on the side.

<u>Grilled Chicken Quesadilla</u>
Serves 2

2 sprouted grain tortillas
1 whole skinless chicken breast
2 cupped hands of canned black beans, drained rinsed
3 ounces goat cheese, crumbled
Chopped red onion to taste
Chopped green pepper to taste
1 tablespoon grated lemon zest
1 tablespoon lime zest
1/4 teaspoon chili powder
1/4 teaspoon cumin
3 tablespoons olive oil
1/4 teaspoon black pepper
1/4 cup fresh chopped cilantro
Juice from one freshly squeezed lemon
Juice from one freshly squeezed lime

1/2 pound fresh asparagus
2 Tablespoons of olive oil
Sea salt
Black pepper

Directions:
Make marinade in a small bowl by whisking together lemon zest, lime zest, 1 tablespoon olive oil, lemon juice and lime juice. Place chicken breast in zip lock bag with marinade and shake to coat. Let marinate at room temperature for 30 minutes turning bag occasionally. Cook chicken on grill over medium heat until well browned and cooked through. Cut into small bite size pieces. In medium skillet, heat 2 tablespoons of oil over medium heat. Add onion and peppers. Sauté, stirring, until soft (about 5 minutes). Add beans, chili powder, cumin, black pepper and 1/2 cup water. Cook, stirring occasionally until most of the water has evaporated.

Spread black bean mixture from skillet over a tortilla. Scatter goat cheese, cilantro and chicken over the tortilla with bean mixture. Place another tortilla on top. Place quesadilla in large skillet lightly coated with olive oil and cook over medium heat for approximately two minutes. Flip to the other side and cook an additional 1 1/2 minutes. Serve topped with fresh guacamole if desired. Enjoy with roasted asparagus on the side.

Preheat oven to 400 degrees F. Place asparagus on a baking sheet, drizzle with olive oil and toss to coat completely. Spread asparagus in a single layer and sprinkle with salt and pepper to taste. Roast for 25 minutes. Enjoy warm.

Sautéed Chicken over Brown Rice
Serves 2

1 boneless, skinless chicken breast
1/4 cup sliced green peppers
1/4 cup sliced red peppers
1/4 cup sliced sweet onions
1/4 cup sliced olives
3 cloves pressed garlic
1 tablespoon olive oil

Handful of freshly sliced pineapple (bite size pieces)
1 tablespoon of plain or honey Greek yogurt

Directions:
Cook brown rice according to rice or rice cooker instructions. Preheat olive oil in deep skillet. Add onions, peppers and garlic. Sauté over medium heat until peppers and onions are tender. Remove onion, garlic and pepper mixture from pan and set aside. Cook chicken breast in same pan until well browned and fully cooked through. Remove chicken from pan and slice into 1/4 inch thick pieces. Serve over brown rice topped with onion, pepper and garlic mixture and sliced olives. Enjoy with pineapple in Greek yogurt on the side.

Baked Salmon with Steamed Vegetables
Serves 6 – Salmon Recipe Courtesy Gailann Greene

1 (2 to 2 1/2-pound) salmon fillet
1/4 cup olive oil
1 lemon
1/4 teaspoon sea salt
1/4 teaspoon cracked Szechwan pepper

1/2 cup fresh dill

6 hand-sized portions of fresh mixed vegetables

Directions:
Preheat oven to 400 degrees Fahrenheit. Place a sheet of parchment paper on the bottom of a roasting pan and drizzle paper with olive oil. Place salmon on the paper skin side down and drizzle with olive oil, followed by a squeeze of fresh lemon, sea salt, Szechwan pepper and dill. Bake until done, salmon will be flaky (approximately 12-15 minutes). Steam mixed vegetables according to steamer instructions and season to taste. Serve warm.

Vegetable Curry over Brown Rice
Serves 4

1 1/2 teaspoons olive oil
1 cup chopped broccoli
1 cup chopped cauliflower
1/2 cup sliced yellow onion
1/2 cup sliced red pepper
1/2 cup sliced green pepper
2 teaspoons curry powder
1 cup vegetable broth
1/4 teaspoon salt
2 cups chickpeas
1/4 cup chopped fresh cilantro
1/2 cup unsalted cashews

Directions:
Cook brown rice according to package or rice cooker directions. Preheat olive oil in large skillet over medium heat. Add broccoli, cauliflower, onion, peppers and curry powder. Cook 1 to 3 minutes, stirring constantly. Add broth, salt and chickpeas. Bring to a boil. Cover and reduce heat, simmer 10 minutes or until vegetables are tender, stirring occasionally. Serve over brown rice topped with cilantro and cashews.

Scott A. Johnson

Tilapia and Quinoa
Serves 4

1 cup quinoa
2 teaspoons olive oil
1 yellow onion, chopped
2 cloves garlic, minced
1 14-ounce can vegetable broth
Juice of one fresh lime
1/2 cup fresh cilantro, chopped
1/4 teaspoon salt

4 tilapia fillets
2 tablespoon olive oil
1 tablespoon fresh lemon juice
1 pinch dired basil
1 pinch dried oregano

4 handfuls mixed vegetables (carrots, cauliflower and broccoli)
2 tablespoons olive oil
Sea Salt
Black Pepper

Directions:
Quinoa: Toast quinoa in large dry skillet over medium heat for 3 to 5 minutes, stirring often. Place in fine strainer and rinse thoroughly. Heat oil in large saucepan over medium heat. Sautee onion until softened. Add garlic and cook stirring constantly for 1 minute. Add the quinoa and broth. Bring to a simmer. Reduce heat and allow to simmer covered until most of the liquid is absorbed, about 20 minutes. Add cilantro, salt and lime juice and fluff with fork.

Tilapia: Heat 2 tablespoons olive oil in large skillet over medium heat. Sprinkle both side of each tilapia fillet with lemon juice, basil and oregano. Place fillets in heated skillet without allowing them to touch. Sear fillets for 2 to 3 minutes on each side, until browned and flaky on the inside. Serve over quinoa.

Roasted Vegetables:

Preheat oven to 400 degrees F. Place vegetables in a baking sheet, drizzle with olive oil and toss to coat completely. Spread vegetables in a single layer and sprinkle with salt and pepper to taste. Roast for 25 minutes. Enjoy warm.

Baked Sweet Potato with Side Blueberry, Apple, Pecan Salad
Serves 4

4 sweet potatoes
4 tablespoons butter
Cinnamon to taste

4 to 6 handfuls of mixed greens
1 granny smith apple, diced
2 cupped hands of blueberries
1 cupped hand of pecans, chopped
1/4 cup blue cheese crumbles
Raspberry vinaigrette dressing from pg. 52-53

Directions:
Create salad by placing mixed greens, apples and blueberries in large bowl. Add dressing to taste and toss to mix well. Add blue cheese crumbles and serve.

Preheat oven to 450 degrees. Scrub and clean sweet potatoes and dry with paper towel. Poke several holes in each sweet potato. Place sweet potatoes on cookie sheet. Cook for 30 minutes then turn over and cook another 30 minutes. Cool slightly then cut open and place one tablespoon butter in middle. Sprinkle with cinnamon to taste. Enjoy.

Herb Roasted Salmon, New Potatoes and Side Mixed Greens Salad
Serves 6 – Salmon Recipe Courtesy Gailann Greene

1 (1 1/2 to 2-pound) salmon fillet
1/4 cup olive oil
1 lemon
1/4 teaspoon sea salt
1/4 teaspoon cracked Szechwan pepper
1/2 cup fresh dill

6-8 new potatoes

Scott A. Johnson

2 tablespoons olive oil
2 cloves garlic minced
1 teaspoon fresh rosemary
1/4 teaspoon sea salt
1/4 teaspoon pepper

4 to 6 handfuls of mixed greens
Balsamic vinaigrette dressing

Directions:
Preheat oven to 450 degrees Fahrenheit. Wash potatoes and cut in half. Place potatoes in mixing bowl and add olive oil, garlic, rosemary, salt and pepper. Toss until potatoes are well covered. Spread potatoes out on a single layer of a baking pan. Roast for until potatoes are thoroughly cooked and browned (approximately 40 minutes).

Add salmon to oven when potatoes have approximately 15 minutes left. Place a sheet of parchment paper on the bottom of a roasting pan and drizzle paper with olive oil. Place salmon on the paper skin side down and drizzle with olive oil, followed by a squeeze of fresh lemon, sea salt, Szechwan pepper and dill. Bake until done, salmon will be flaky (approximately 12-15 minutes).

Place salmon and potato portions on dinner plate. Add handful of mixed greens and top with balsamic vinaigrette. Enjoy while salmon and potatoes are still hot.

Kamut Pasta and Pasta Sauce
Serves 6

12 ounces kamut pasta
1 tablespoon butter
8 small tomatoes, diced
1/3 cup chopped basil
1 1/4 teaspoon olive oil
1 clove garlic, chopped
1/2 cup black beans, drained, rinsed and blended finely in a blender

16 ounces of fresh green beans, trimmed
1 tablespoon olive oil
2 teaspoons shredded parmesan

68

Sea salt to taste
Pepper to taste

Directions:
Preheat oven to 425 degrees F. Place green beans on baking sheet and drizzle olive oil on them. Season with salt and pepper if desired. Toss to evenly coat. Spread them evenly on baking sheet. Bake 8 minutes. Shake pan to turn over and bake an additional 7 minutes. Remove from pan and sprinkle with cheese.

Melt butter in large skillet over medium heat. Add tomatoes to butter and cook until they start to fall apart. Add basil, olive oil, black beans and salt and pepper if desired. Simmer for 5 minutes then add garlic and simmer an additional 5 minutes stirring occasionally. Leave sauce on lowest heat setting to keep warm while cooking pasta. Cook pasta according to package directions. Serve sauce over pasta, with a side of roasted green beans.

Salsa Chicken and Tortilla Salad
Serves 6

2 large boneless, skinless chicken breasts
1 1/2 cup favorite salsa
1/4 cup honey
1 teaspoon cumin
1 clove garlic, minced
1/2 cup Italian dressing
6 sprouted grain tortillas
1 head Romaine lettuce
12 ounces cooked black beans
2 cups brown rice

Dressing:
1 package ranch dressing mix (prepared according to package directions)
1 tomatillo
Juice from one lime
1 clove garlic, minced
1 jalapeno pepper
1/2 bunch of cilantro

Scott A. Johnson

Directions:
Place chicken breasts in crock pot and cover with salsa, honey, cumin, garlic and Italian dressing. Cook for 6 to 8 hours on low or 3 to 5 hours on high. Prepare rice according to package or rice cooker instructions. Prepare dressing by combing dressing ingredients in a blender and blend until smooth. Adjust jalapeno, lime juice and cilantro to taste. Shred chicken. Place tortilla in single size serving bowl and top with beans, rice, lettuce and chicken. Enjoy with dressing on top or on the side.

Made in the USA
Lexington, KY
13 September 2014